A THEORETICAL GUIDE TO
ESPORTS
NUTRITION

ANDRÉ BAUMANN

ISBNs: 978-82-691601-0-9 (paperback)
978-82-691601-1-6 (ebook)

First printing, 2019.

www.gamersperformance.com

ABBREVIATIONS

5-HT	Serotonin
ALA	Alpha-linolenic acid
BCAA	Branched-chain amino acids
BMR	Basal metabolic rate
BR	Battle royale
DHA	Docosahexaenoic acid
DIT	Diet-induced thermogenesis
DP	Degree of polymerization
DV	Daily value
EAA	Essential Amino acids
ED	Energy drinks
EE	Energy expenditure
EPA	Eicosapentaenoic acid
FAO	Food and Agricultural Organization of the United Nations
FPS	First-person shooter
G	Gram(s)
GI	Glycemic index
GL	Glycemic load
Kcal	Kilocalories
LAN	Local area network
LDL	Low-density lipoproteins
Mg	Milligrams
MOBA	Multiplayer online battle arena
MPS	Muscle protein synthesis
MUFA	Monounsaturated fatty acids
N-3 VLCPUFA	Very long-chain omega-3 PUFA
NASCAR	National Association for Stock Car Auto Racing
NREM	Non-rapid eye movement

NSP	Non-starch polysaccharides
PA	Physical activity
PAL	Physical activity level
PDCAAS	Protein digestibility-corrected amino acid score
PUFA	Polyunsaturated fatty acids
REM	Rapid eye movement
RMR	Resting metabolic rate
SFA	Saturated fatty acids
TDEE	Total daily energy expenditure
TFA	Trans fatty acids
Trp	Tryptophan
USD	United States dollar
VLDL	Very low-density lipoproteins

TABLE OF CONTENTS

PREFACE

One thing came to my mind as the popularity of esports grew and the players became well-paid athletes – *if they are athletes, they need to eat well to perform.* In every sport, athletes need both quality and quantity training. They facilitate this by eating and drinking healthy and getting enough rest. The same principles should apply to esports athletes. Also, someone needs to convey this information. This book aims to deliver evidence-based information tailored to esports athletes, with practical recommendations for each topic.

My experience goes beyond my academic studies or work experience. I used to be an esports athlete nicknamed "SlickSilver" in Counter-Strike 1.6, back in 2004. My team, Catch Gamer, was probably one of the first Norwegian teams to have signed contracts with our sponsors. We won most national championships and performed well internationally. Just before Catch Gamer won the Cyberathlete Professional League tournament in Turkey, I decided to quit the team to focus on my studies and getting my academic degree. I finished my master's degree in nutrition at the University of Oslo several years later and got a job at the Norwegian Olympic Sports Center, working as a nutritionist. I got to work with world-class Olympic athletes – a dream job for me as a nutritionist interested in competitive sports.

I hope the combination of my academic and empirical background will help those of you who aspire to be a better player – whether you are a "casual" gamer or an esports athlete.

ESPORTS AND ESPORTS ATHLETES

During the last decade, electronic sports, also known as esports, have gained immense popularity. The number of competitive games, players, and teams has increased, along with public interest in esports. There are political discussions regarding esports' position as an Olympic sport or whether it should have its own Olympics. Huge financial investments are made in teams, players, and products. A few companies have also started producing dietary supplements just for improving gaming performance. There is no doubt that esports is a competitive scene with massive interest from both the community and the public, with much financial power behind it and the broad recruitment of new players. Gaming, in general, is for most people accessible, with the equipment cost being a one-time investment, at least for a few years. After that, it is arguably up to the individual how far they want to go – remain a casual gamer or move to the next level, an esports professional.

What separates the semi-professional from the professional players is the same factor as for athletes in other sports – the capacity to work on the details that impact the sport the athletes are playing. These details could be anything from sleep to physical or mental training or nutrition. In this book, it will be discussed how one can achieve going from semi-professional to professional esports player with nutrition as a tool.

DEFINING ESPORTS

Esports is the official terminology for "professional video gaming," which refers to the instance where players are playing against each other – either as individuals or in teams – in a competition. This definition is arguably a somewhat inadequate definition of esports, with a more proper definition proposed as "organized video game competitions" [1]. Esports is still in its infancy, but it is becoming highly popular, and the popularity will most likely increase in the years to come. As of March 2019, more than 60 colleges have esports programs recognized by the National Association of Collegiate Esports (NAC Esports), and this number will probably grow[2; 3].

During the last few years, the number of players, teams, and competitions and the amount of prize money have skyrocketed due to the popularity of the genre. By 2019, over 292 million people will be watching esports[4], and it is estimated that by 2022, over 600 million people will watch esports, with almost 300 million being frequent viewers. Compared to 2018, this is nearly a 50% increase in only four years[5]. The most popular games in esports at the moment are League of Legends, Dota 2, Counter-Strike: Global Offensive, Overwatch, Fortnite Battle Royale, PlayerUnknown's Battlegrounds, Tom Clancy's Rainbow Six Siege, Hearthstone and Call of Duty. The popularity varies between the games in terms of both player base and spectators, but all of the games mentioned above have large tournaments with recognizable prize money. These games can be categorized into first-person shooters (FPS), Battle Royale (BR), and multiplayer online battle arena (MOBA).

NUTRITION AND PHYSICAL HEALTH IN GAMERS AND ESPORTS ATHLETES

Trying to create evidence-based nutritional advice for esports players is not easy. Only a few studies have been done on esports, and most of the reviews explore the behavioral or psychological factors[6; 7; 8; 9; 10]. At a Local Area Network (LAN), one can observe that many of the attendees are consuming unhealthy food and drink items. The usual food and drink products at these events range from fast food, candy, sodas, and energy drinks – to the occasional healthy sandwich. These food choices are the standard for a lot of the "casual" gamers and even a few of the professional ones. Some of the professional players have a good training regime and a dietary plan they follow, but they are far from the majority. Unfortunately, there are no studies done on this specific population regarding dietary pattern. According to Statista, the estimated number of gamers at the end of 2017 was approximately 2,2 billion[11]. The age group ranges from 10 to 35 years old, which represents a total of 65% of both men and women characterized as gamers worldwide[12]. This age group also includes the esports professional players, who are usually between 15 and the early- to mid-30s.

A recent study on esports athletes from nine universities across Canada and the USA shed some light on their current health habits. Anonymous electronic surveys were sent out to these players, inquiring about gaming and lifestyle habits, as well as musculoskeletal complaints. Before competitions, the esports athletes practiced between five and ten hours a day, with fifteen percent reporting they sat three hours or more without standing or taking a break. Forty percent said that they did not do any physical activity regularly. Regarding pain or fatigue, eye fatigue was most prominent, followed by back and neck pain, with 52% and 41% acknowledging this, respectively. Approximately one-third of the athletes also reported both hand and wrist pain. Interestingly, only 2% of these players sought medical attention[9].

Gamers and esports athletes are found all over the world and in different socio-economic classes. A typical diet pattern for many people around the world is the "Western diet," which is known for a high intake of saturated and omega-6 fatty acids, a high salt intake, reduced omega-3 fatty acids, and an overconsumption of refined sugar[13]. Chronic overuse of this type of diet can cause morbidity and mortality. Damage to the kidneys and heart, obesity, diabetes, cancer, metabolic syndrome, and adverse effects on the immune system are only a few of the consequences[14]. It is likely that some of these gamers and athletes follow this type of diet; in addition, this is a population that sits for many hours a day[9].

THE INDIVIDUALIZED APPROACH

The guidelines in this book are based on studies done on subject populations resembling the esports athletes, but as already mentioned, there are very few studies done on nutrition in the esports population. However, one of the most important aspects of nutrition is the individualized approach. For optimal results, one must take into account individual variations. We each have a slightly different internal make-up – some have intolerances or allergies, and we have different gut bacteria. Also, we have different food preferences, activity levels, and general lifestyles. Everything has to be accounted for when trying to optimize nutritional routines, which is why help from professionals is necessary for every athlete trying to achieve top results.

NUTRITIONAL DEMANDS IN ESPORTS

Currently, there are no guidelines for esports athletes regarding nutrition. The goal for the coming chapters is to discuss and create some guidelines that can improve both health and performance for esports athletes. It is important to acknowledge that health and performance affect each other. Therefore, much of the nutritional advice will also have its foundation in good health. With better health, one can prolong the esports career of the athlete, as well as increase the performance.

ENERGY REQUIREMENTS AND DAILY ENERGY INTAKE

Individual energy requirements are based on energy demands. If one exercises a lot or has an active lifestyle, one's energy requirements will increase. People who are undernourished or obese might, in some periods, choose to have a higher or lower energy intake to either gain or lose weight. However, long-term energy balance is the most beneficial state. The total daily energy expenditure (TDEE), the number of calories you use per day, is based on the following three components[15]:

1. Basal metabolic rate (BMR) or resting metabolic rate (RMR)
2. Diet-induced thermogenesis (DIT)
3. Physical activity (PA)

The gold standard for measuring TDEE in a free-living context is a technique called doubly labeled water. However, calculating a precise measure of PA is very difficult considering all the variables and complexity. Usually, a value for physical activity level (PAL) is chosen when estimating the active energy expenditure[16]. The PAL values usually range from 1,40 to 2,40[16], and the Food and

Agricultural Organization of the United Nations (FAO) has listed several examples of PAL values based on different lifestyles, from a sedentary lifestyle up to a vigorously active lifestyle[17]. These values are multiplied by the RMR to get an estimate for the TDEE. In the western diet, the TDEE is often lower than the energy intake. This lower energy intake will result in a weight increase, which can lead to obesity and increased morbidity and mortality[18].

The RMR represents the energy expenditure (EE) at rest in a thermo-neutral environment while having fasted, and typically results in a higher EE than BMR, since it is measured under less strict conditions[16]. One of the most critical factors that can affect RMR is body composition. Body composition is adjustable with diet and exercise intervention. For instance, increasing the amount of muscle mass will increase the amount of active metabolic tissue, resulting in an increased RMR[19; 20].

PRACTICAL RECOMMENDATIONS FOR DAILY ENERGY INTAKE FOR ESPORTS ATHLETES

In esports, which have a relatively low physical activity level, not exceeding the TDEE is important. An increased body weight (fat mass) over time will be detrimental for both health and performance. To counter this, it is essential that one eats a healthy and balanced diet while doing regular physical activity. A combination of strength and cardiovascular training will ensure the benefits of both training categories. Getting professional help with estimating the TDEE might be a good idea if an esports athlete is considering doing weight regulation (i.e., planning to reduce or gain weight). It is essential to have a qualified opinion when estimating the PAL values, to get as accurate a TDEE as possible. Getting help from a nutritionist or dietitian will ease the process and probably save a lot of time and frustration.

MACRONUTRIENTS

Macronutrients are the energy-giving substances in our food; they comprise proteins, fats, and carbohydrates. Alcohol and dietary fiber also give us calories but in a different amount than the macronutrients mentioned above. For esports athletes, the distribution of these macronutrients is vital for both performance and health.

PROTEIN AND AMINO ACIDS

STRUCTURE AND FUNCTION

Dietary protein provides us with 4 kcal per gram. The protein we get through our food is digested and used for multiple purposes. Some of these processes include building muscle tissue through muscle protein synthesis, structural function, membranes, enzymes, and hormones. In the intestines, the proteins we consume are broken down into smaller molecules called amino acids. These amino acids provide nitrogen, hydrocarbon skeletons, and sulfur. No other nutrients can replace these components. Most proteins contain 20 different amino acids, of which 9 are essential and must be included in the diet. The remaining amino acids can be synthesized endogenously. Table 1 below shows these 20 amino acids and which of them are essential amino acids (EAA) and branched-chain amino acids (BCAA)[21]. BCAAs have been associated with increased muscle growth; however, recent studies show that BCAAs alone as a supplement do not augment muscle growth[22; 23].

Table 1. The table shows the 20 different amino acids found in familiar protein sources, as well as the essential amino acids and branched-chained amino acids.

Amino Acid	Essential Amino Acid	Branched-chain amino acid
Alanine	No	No
Arginine	No	No
Asparagine	No	No
Aspartic acid	No	No
Cysteine	No	No
Glutamine	No	No
Glutamic acid	No	No
Glycine	No	No
Histidine	Yes	No
Isoleucine	Yes	Yes
Leucine	Yes	Yes
Lysine	Yes	No
Methionine	Yes	No
Phenylalanine	Yes	No
Proline	No	No
Serine	No	No
Threonine	Yes	No
Tryptophan	Yes	No
Tyrosine	No	No
Valine	Yes	Yes

(21)

Proteins have different levels of structure, with the primary structure being the sequence of amino acids in the polypeptide chain. The forces that hold this chain together are polypeptide bonds. The secondary structure of a protein refers to the folded structures that form within a polypeptide due to interactions between the backbone of the atoms. Two of the most common conformations are the α-helix and the β-pleated sheet. The tertiary structure of a protein is the three-dimensional structure of mono- and multimeric protein molecules, in which the chains are folded to compact structures stabilized by disulfide bridges, hydrogen bonds, and van der Waals forces. Finally, the quaternary structure is the non-covalent relation of proteins due to the hydrogen bonds and van der Waals forces mentioned above[21].

PROTEIN QUALITY

There are several methods used to rank the quality of protein. The first method, biological value (BV), calculates the nitrogen used for tissue formation divided by the nitrogen absorbed from the food. BV provides us with a measurement of how efficiently the body uses the protein consumed in the diet, which means that a protein with a high value supplies us with a lot of EAA. The second method, net protein utilization, is akin to the BV method, except it directly measures absorbed nitrogen retention. The main difference between these two methods of measuring nitrogen retention is that NPU calculates this from nitrogen ingested, while BV derives this from nitrogen absorbed[24]. Finally, there is the protein digestibility-corrected amino acid score (PDCAAS), which scores the protein quality based on the limiting EAA in the protein compared to a reference protein, multiplied by the ability to digest the protein. PDCAAS is currently the most accepted method of evaluating protein quality. However, there are discussions regarding its shortcomings[24; 25; 26].

GENERAL RECOMMENDATIONS

In this section, only recommendations for healthy adults (aged 18 – 65 years) are discussed. The recommended intake of protein in the diet is usually in grams per kilo bodyweight (g/kg), but some recommendations are based on the percentage of daily caloric intake. The recommendation based on the percentage of daily caloric intake varies with PAL, with a lower PAL having a higher recommendation for protein. A PAL of 1,6 has a recommendation of 10% of the energy coming from protein, while a PAL of 1,4 has a recommendation of 20% of the energy coming from protein. In summary, the recommended level of protein coming from the total energy intake is from 10% to 20%, which corresponds to 0,8 to 1,5 grams of protein per kilo bodyweight per day[15].

The requirement for most people is based on nitrogen balance; however, the methodological pitfall of this method is being discussed[27]. The recommended dietary intake for a healthy adult is 0,83 grams protein per kg body weight per day, with a PDCAAS of 1. This recommendation comes from an estimated average requirement of 0,66 grams per kilo bodyweight per day[28]. For athletes, the dietary guidelines are based on muscle protein synthesis (MPS). For example, strength and power athletes require a higher protein intake than endurance athletes. This increased demand is due to an increased rate of MPS post workout, lasting up to approximately 48 hours[29]. Table 2 illustrates the recommendations for protein for different populations[30].

Table 2. The table illustrates the protein recommendation for different types of population.

Population	The recommendation, grams per kg
Sedentary	0,8
Endurance athletes	1,2 – 1,6
Strength and power training	1,4 – 1,7

[30]

The most important part is to reach the daily protein requirements, but the distribution of protein per meal also seems to play an essential part in stimulating maximal MPS. Aiming for 20-25 grams of high-quality protein, or 0,24 to 0,30 grams per kilo bodyweight per meal, seems to be the optimal range, assuming the protein source is of good quality. Choosing high-quality protein most likely ensures that the metabolic trigger for MPS, the amino acid leucine, is available in sufficient amounts. Consuming enough proteins containing leucine post exercise might be the most optimal strategy for increasing MPS in this acute phase. For experienced weight-trained individuals with a high lean body mass and a low body fat mass in a weight reduction phase, a higher protein intake per day can be advocated to help prevent loss of muscle mass[26; 31]. Based on the current evidence, there are no upper intake levels of protein[15]. However, increasing the protein intake beyond the recommendation mentioned above might result in a sub-optimal diet composition as it reduces the intake of carbohydrates, fiber, and fat and the micronutrients corresponding to these components.

FOOD SOURCES

Dietary proteins are found in most food items we consume, of both plant and animal origin. However, the quality of protein can vary a lot. Usually, protein from animals has a higher quality, meaning it has a better amino acid composition. These proteins contain all of the 20 amino acids. Some high-quality protein sources are meat, fish, poultry, milk, eggs, and cheese[27].

Good sources of plant proteins include cereal grains, legumes, and nuts[32]. Plant-based foods are the primary source of protein globally, accounting for 57% of the daily protein intake, followed by meat at 18%[33].

<u>PRACTICAL RECOMMENDATIONS FOR ESPORTS ATHLETES</u>

The protein recommendation depends on the lifestyle of the player. Some esports players do rigorous strength training 4-6 times a week, which may total 6 to 10 hours per week. For these players, there is a higher demand for protein in the diet to facilitate optimal recovery and muscle growth. These players should try to achieve 1,4-1,7 g protein per kilo bodyweight.

On the other hand, a player who is sedentary, with little to no physical activity, probably does not need more than 0,8 g protein per kg body weight. For an 80-kg athlete who is not doing any physical activity, the protein requirement will amount to 64 g protein per day. For an athlete who weighs the same but has heavy strength training several times a week, the requirement will probably be in the area of 112-136 g protein per day. This example shows a considerable difference in protein requirement which will influence what type of food to select for each meal. In summary, the guidelines for protein intake should be tailored to each athlete – depending on the amount, the type, and the intensity of the physical activity.

Aside from the protein recommendations per day, there are other factors to take into account. The protein should be of high quality, as well as evenly distributed throughout the day. Lean protein sources are preferable, and variation is essential in order to get all the necessary micronutrients. In summary, for an esports player the following is most important:

1. Adjust the daily protein intake according to the lifestyle – heavy strength or cardiovascular training requires more protein than a sedentary lifestyle.

2. Protein intake should range between 0,8 and 1,7 grams per kilo bodyweight per day.

3. Distribute the protein evenly in meals throughout the day.

4. Protein quality should be high in every meal, the best protein sources being eggs, meat, poultry, fish, and dairy products.

FATS AND FATTY ACIDS

STRUCTURE AND FUNCTION

The fat one eats in foods are vital to the human body. Different types of fat have different types of function in our body. Common to all types of fat is the great potential as energy storage in our body. There are different types of fat; some go hard in the refrigerator, and some are liquid. This consistency is related to what type of fatty acid the food item contains, and it is essential to know the difference between these types and what they do in our body, in order to choose what is best for health and performance.

The fats naturally existing are usually a combination of triglycerides, which are made up of one molecule of glycerol esterified with three fatty acid molecules. One gram of dietary fat gives approximately 9 kcal[21]. Usually, these fatty acids contain from 16 to 18 carbon atoms. The effects the different fatty acids have on our body depend on multiple factors, e.g., carbon chain length, the degree of saturation, and the number, structure, and position of the double bonds. These fatty acids have generally been divided into different groups: saturated fatty acids (SFA), monounsaturated fatty acids (MUFA), and polyunsaturated fatty acids (PUFA). MUFAs contain only one double bond, while PUFAs have between two and six double bonds[15]. Table 3 shows the different categories of fatty acids and some of their everyday dietary food sources[21; 34; 35].

Table 3. The table shows our three main dietary fat categories, as well as some of the common dietary fats found in each of these categories. Additionally, it shows different food items from which we can get these dietary fats, as well as the usual amount represented in the diet.

Dietary fat category	Common dietary fats	Food items	Percentage of daily fat intake
Triglycerides	Linoleic acid, oleic acid, stearic acid, α-linolenic acid, docosahexaenoic acid, eicosapentaenoic acid	Oils, nuts, eggs, avocado, fish	≤ 95
Phospholipids	Phosphatidylcholine, phosphatidylserine, phosphatidylinositol	Eggs, organ and lean meats, fish, shellfish, oilseeds, cereal grains	1-10
Cholesterol	Cholesterol*	Eggs, cheese, organ meats	<1**

* Cholesterol has different binding proteins for transportation and absorption, more commonly known as very low-density lipoproteins (VLDL), low-density lipoproteins (LDL), and high-density lipoproteins.

**The average intake of cholesterol in U.S. adults is between 200 and 350 mg per day, which equates to less than 1% of the total daily fat intake per day[21; 34; 35].

The functions of fatty acids include being components of lipids and cell membranes and working as an energy substrate[36]. It has been established for quite some time that an increased intake of MUFA or PUFA at the expense of SFA reduces the risk of coronary heart disease, as does a lower intake of trans fatty acids (TFAs)[37]. Fish or seafood contains very long-chain omega-3 PUFA (n-3 VLCPUFA), which have important functions in our body, and a high intake of n-3 VLCPUFAs will lower plasma triglycerides, blood pressure, and heart rate, as well as inhibiting pro-inflammatory processes[38; 39; 40; 41; 42]. The effects of n-3 VLCPUFAs on the brain are still unclear when supplemented above the recommended range, though there might be benefits from some of these essential fatty acids, with the proposed benefits being largest with docosahexaenoic acid (DHA)[43].

COGNITIVE FUNCTION

Current reviews and meta-analyses are inconclusive about the effect of supplementation of omega-3 fatty acids on cognitive performance[44; 45; 46]. The review indicating an improved cognitive function proposed this effect only when the supplementation was with low doses of omega-3 fatty acids (<1,73 g/day); there were no benefits at higher dosages[44]. One of the meta-analyses included only participants with an age above 60 years or a diagnosis of a condition (e.g., memory complaints, Alzheimer's disease, mild cognitive impairment), or both[45]. These subject groups might not be too applicable for our purpose. Finally, the last concluded that it was unclear whether n-3 LCPUFA resulted in any cognition improvement in young and healthy adults. Only one of the studies in this review indicated an improved cognitive performance for this subject group[47].

The studies included in the reviews and meta-analyses mentioned above vary in the number of participants, gender, age, health status, duration of intervention, supplementation protocol, and method of assessing cognitive function. Also, controlling the diet is essential, as study participants might already have a high intake of omega-3 fatty acids in their diet, confounding the results of the supplementation protocol. For esports athletes, future research should be directed at young and healthy individuals in the age group corresponding to these athletes, mostly from teenagers up to the mid-30s. Regarding the methods of use, tailoring specific tests for esports athletes should be feasible.

GENERAL RECOMMENDATIONS

It is important to know how much fat one should have in the diet, both for health and performance. Too much fat can increase the total energy intake in the diet, as well as the potential for a lot of unhealthy fat types, such as saturated and trans fatty acids. Too little fat and one might miss out on essential fatty acids and a lot of essential vitamins, such as vitamin A, D, E, and K. Vitamin D might be of particular importance for esports athletes, as they might have a lower vitamin D status due to less sun exposure. The recommended intake of vitamin D is 10 μg per day for adults, which is usually covered by ingesting a regular fish oil supplement[15].

FAO considers that the acceptable macronutrient distribution ranges between 20% and 35% of the total daily energy intake. Total fat intake should be higher than 15% of the total daily energy intake, which is the minimum amount to ensure that one gets enough essential fatty acids and energy. For individuals with a moderate physical activity level, 30% of the energy intake is recommended, and for those with a high level of physical activity, up to 35%. The amount of SFA is proposed to be no more than 10% of the daily energy intake and TFA no more than 1%. The range of PUFA should be between 6% and 11%, and the remaining fatty acids should come from MUFA, which will vary according to the intake of the other fatty acids. The formulae for MUFA recommendations will then be MUFA = total fat intake (E%) – SFA – PUFA – TFA[48]. The Nordic Nutrition Recommendations from 2012 have the following recommendations for fat based on the total daily energy intake: SFA intake below 10%, TFA as low as possible, MUFA between 10% and 20%, PUFA between 5% and 10%, and a total fat intake of between 25% and 40%. For dietary planning purposes, NNR 2012 recommends a middle range value of 32-33% of the daily total energy intake[15].

The National Institute of Health has the following guidelines for ages 9 and older for omega-3 fatty acids[49]:

Table 4. Adequate intakes (AIs) of omega-3 fatty acids

Age in years	Male, grams	Female (non-pregnant/non-lactating), grams
9 – 13*	1,2	1
14+*	1,6	1,1

*As alpha-linolenic acid (ALA).[49]

However, FAO has concluded that 0,5-0,6% of the daily energy intake should be the minimum requirement for ALA. The total omega-3 fatty acid intake (ALA; EPA and DHA) can lie between 0,5% and 2% of the total energy intake. For adult males and non-pregnant/non-lactating females, the minimum intake of EPA is set at 0,250 gram per day plus DHA. There is a general agreement that up to 3 grams of n-3 LCPUFA per day is safe to consume[48]. The Nordic Nutrition Recommendations (NNR 2012) recommend that from 2 years old, at least 1% of the daily energy intake should come from omega-3 fatty acids. Preferably up to 3% of the daily energy intake should come from essential fatty acids, e.g., ALA, with at least 0,5% of the daily intake being ALA[15].

FOOD SOURCES

Most food items contain fatty acids to some degree. Some of these foods contain more SFA, while others contain MUFA or PUFA. What differs in most products is the ratio of the fatty acids. As already discussed, it is most beneficial, from a general health perspective, to have a low amount of SFA in the diet, with the most substantial amount of fatty acids coming from MUFA and PUFA.

The typical fat sources containing a lot of SFA are solid at room temperature. This solidifying is usually an indicator of fat sources that one wants to avoid. Examples of these fat sources are butter, fats from red meat (pork, lamb, and beef), coconut butter, and milk fat. Typical food items in which one can find these fats are cakes, cookies, donuts, pastries, sausages, ice cream, fries, pizza, and other similar products. These are the typical foods one should stay away from – not just because of their unhealthy fatty acids but because of other factors such as high energy density, low nutrient density, and sugar content.

The primary sources of PUFA and some of the earlier-mentioned essential fatty acids such as alpha-linolenic acid are usually fish and fish oils. Fish such as mackerel, salmon, and trout are rich in these omega-3 fatty acids that are important for our health. Other sources of PUFA are soft margarine and vegetable oils[15].

When it comes to MUFA, a lot of different food items contain these fatty acids. However, the foods containing the most MUFA are various nuts, oils, avocado, and animal products. Oils have the highest density of MUFA, followed by nuts, avocado, pork, eggs, and bacon. Table 5 below shows the ratio and fatty acid composition of some of the food items mentioned above.

Table 5. The table illustrates the fatty acid composition of different food items in grams.

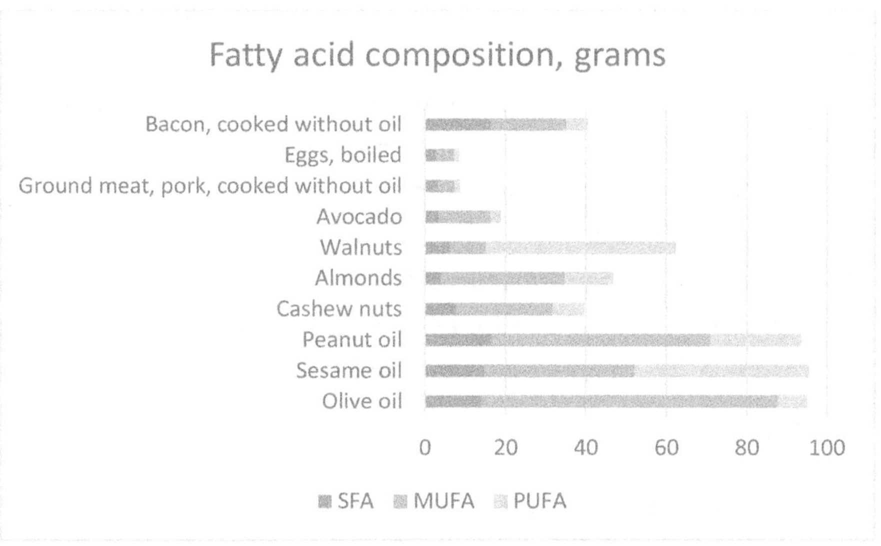

Data obtained from www.matvaretabellen.no, with the search names matching the names displayed in this table. All data is estimated from 100 grams of an edible food item. Data collected 31 January 2019[50].

PRACTICAL RECOMMENDATIONS FOR ESPORTS ATHLETES

The lack of scientific research on esports players as a population, as well as the performance effect of fats on sports comparable to esports, make the guidelines for fatty acid intake vague when it comes to performance. The most important thing is that one ensures the following:

1. Fatty fish for dinner twice a week

2. Fish oil as a supplement with vitamin D every day

3. A handful of different unsalted nuts every day

4. Olive oil and avocado used in salads, and margarine on bread

By consuming the recommended amount of fish oil once a day, usually 5 ml, one is also ensuring the minimum requirement for omega-3 fatty acids according to the FAO recommendations. One of the typical fish oil supplements in Norway gives 1,2 grams of omega-3 fatty acids, with 0,6 grams from DHA and 0,4 grams from EPA[51]. Taking fish oil supplements containing vitamin D may also be important, as much time is spent sitting indoors, thus missing out on the best source of vitamin D – sun exposure. However, even though there is limited data on the effect of dietary fat intake on performance, it is essential for health. Eating enough healthy fats will ensure a lot of the essential fatty acids, as well as the fat-soluble vitamins.

CARBOHYDRATES AND DIETARY FIBER

STRUCTURE AND FUNCTION

This macronutrient contributes to a lot of daily energy needs. It is a potent nutrient for high-intensity physical activity, as well as our primary fuel source for the brain. One gram of carbohydrate gives 4 kcal, while one gram of fiber gives approximately 2 kcal. Sugar alcohols give a bit more than fiber, with between 2 and 3 kcal per gram of sugar alcohol[15]. The different types of dietary carbohydrate are defined primarily by their molecular size (degree of polymerization (DP)). Sugars, also called mono- and disaccharides, have 1-2 DP. Different types of mono- and disaccharides are glucose, fructose, galactose, sucrose, lactose, and trehalose. Oligosaccharides have 3-9 DP, for example, maltooligosaccharides. Polysaccharides have 10 or more DP, with the most common subgroup being starch. Table 6 below illustrates the different DP of carbohydrates, as well as the subgroups and components[15; 21; 52; 53].

Table 6. This table illustrates the different carbohydrates according to their degree of polymerization, with the relevant subgroup, most common components, and food sources.

The degree of polymerization (DP)	Subgroup	Components	Common food items
Sugars, 1-2 DP	Monosaccharides	Glucose, galactose, fructose	Fruits, vegetables, honey
	Disaccharides	Sucrose, lactose, trehalose	Chocolate, candy, milk, table sugar
	Polyols	Sorbitol, mannitol	Sugar-free chewing gum
Oligosaccharides, 3 - 9 DP	Maltooligosaccharides	Maltodextrins	Food additives (e.g., sports products)
	Other oligosaccharides	Raffinose, stachyose, fructooligosaccharides	Cereals, fruits, vegetables
Polysaccharides, ≥ 10 DP	Starch	Amylose, amylopectin	Potatoes, bread
	Non-starch polysaccharides	Cellulose, hemicellulose, pectins	Fruits, vegetables

(15; 21; 52; 53)

All these types of carbohydrates can be divided into two broad categories:

1. Digestible carbohydrates
2. Non-digestible carbohydrates

The digestible carbohydrates, also known as glycemic carbohydrates, are absorbed in the small intestine and provide substrates for various body tissues. The glycemic carbohydrates are glucose, fructose, sucrose, lactose, and starch. The non-digestible carbohydrates, also called non-starch polysaccharides (NSP), pass through to the large intestine and assist our colonic microflora. These carbohydrates are the main components of dietary fiber[21].

In western countries, about 50% of dietary fiber comes from cereals, 30-40% from vegetables, 16% from fruits, and the remaining 3% from other minor sources[54]. Table 7 below shows some everyday food items, their total fiber, insoluble fiber, and soluble fiber per 100 gram of edible food source[55].

Table 7. The table shows different food sources and their fiber composition, as well as total fiber. The numbers are based on 100 grams of an edible food item.

Food items	Insoluble fiber	Soluble fiber	Total fiber
Wheat, whole grain	10,2	2,3	12,6
Oats	6,5	3,8	10,3
Green beans	1,4	0,5	1,9
Kidney beans	4,7	1,6	6,3
Potato, without skin	1	0,3	1,3
Beetroot	5,4	2,4	7,8
Tomato, raw	0,8	0,4	1,2
Carrot, raw	3	0,29	3,29
Apple	1,8	0,2	2
Kiwi	2,61	0,8	3,39
Banana	1,2	0,5	1,7
Strawberry	1,3	0,9	2,2
Almonds	10,1	1,1	11,2
Sesame seed	5,89	1,9	7,79
Flaxseed	10,15	12,18	22,33

(55)

BLOOD SUGAR

Carbohydrates are the macronutrient with the most profound effect on blood sugar levels. Depending on several factors, the glycemic index (GI) and glycemic load (GL) of a meal are two of the most discussed factors that contribute to the elevation of blood sugar levels after a meal. The GI tells how significant an impact the food item will have on the blood sugar and is calculated as the area under the blood sugar response curve after 50 grams of glycemic carbohydrate food/the response after the standard (usually glucose or white bread)[21]. For example, a carbohydrate with no dietary fiber, based on mono- or disaccharides, can have a GI of 63 (e.g., Coca Cola)[56]. In contrast, a starch-rich carbohydrate with much dietary fiber might have a GI of 40 (wheat and rye bread)[57]. If one were to eat these two food items in separate meals, with the same amount of total carbohydrate, the energy drink would have more impact on the blood sugar than the whole-grain bread. The result would be higher blood sugar levels from the energy drink than from the bread. The consequence is an increased secretion of insulin to regulate the blood sugar levels towards fasting levels. Other proposed benefits of stable blood sugar levels are better appetite control and mood, as well as a lowered risk of developing maturity-onset diabetes and cardiovascular disease[21]. Well-regulated blood sugar could also be important for athletes engaging in cognitively demanding tasks, such as esports.

The total effect on the blood sugar after a meal is determined by both the GI of the food items consumed and the amount of carbohydrate in the meal. Here is where the concept of GL comes into play; it is the product of the amount of available carbohydrate of the food item, multiplied by the GI of the food, then divided by 100. Hence, the amount of carbohydrate per meal will play a significant role in the blood sugar response after a meal[21].

Apart from GI and GL, there are other factors which have an impact on blood sugar. These – in order of magnitude – are weight reduction and physical activity, dietary fiber, the food matrix (the structure of the food), prebiotics, meal composition, micronutrients, and phytochemicals[58].

COGNITIVE FUNCTION

There have been several studies on refined carbohydrates (simple sugars) and cognitive function, both on the acute and chronic/lifestyle effect. However, the cognitive tests done in these studies might not apply to esports athletes when we evaluate their cognitive performance. For these athletes, further studies are required to assess which type of tests are viable for this subject group when trying to evaluate performance outcomes. Bearing that in mind, it might still be valuable to look at the current data we have on this matter.

Regarding the chronic/lifestyle effect, there seems to be an indication that refined carbohydrates have a deteriorating cognitive effect, particularly in early life. These effects also seem to be unrelated to changes in weight. For acute cognitive performance, there is a discrepancy regarding the potential effects of refined carbohydrates. Some studies support a positive effect, while others show no difference or an adverse effect[59]. However, there are several confounding factors in these studies, making it difficult to compare them, e.g., subject group, carbohydrate type, and composition of the meals. However, since esports gaming requires a high degree of mental strain, usually lasting an hour or more, stable blood sugar might be the best option. In an individualized trial, one can try to manipulate with simple sugars to gain an advantage at the end of a game, but as a general guideline, one should take care not to overdo the sugar intake.

GENERAL RECOMMENDATIONS

Carbohydrates contribute to approximately half of the daily energy intake in the Nordic countries, with the acceptable range being between 45% and 60%. Added sugars account for 10% to 16% and dietary fiber between 25 and 27 grams per approximately 2400 kcal. NNR 2012 also proposes an upper limit of 10% of the total daily energy intake as sugar, as well as a dietary fiber intake of at least 25 grams per day for women and 35 grams per day for men[15]. Other guidelines propose a range between 40% and 75%, with different terminology used for these recommendations[60].

For added sugars, it ranges from 5% up to 25%, but several recommendations are set at an upper limit of 10% of the daily energy intake. Increasing the sugar intake above this range might have unhealthy consequences, as it could lead to a displacement of foods that provide essential micronutrients. Overall, this would lead to a decline in the quality of the diet with potentially negative health consequences[60].

Regarding dietary fiber, most recommendations are above 25 or 30 grams per day. For whole grain products, there is no global consensus for quantitative recommendations[60]. However, in Norway, it is recommended that whole-grain products contribute at least 70 grams to 90 grams per day, as this will help achieve the guidelines for dietary fiber and ensure a higher nutrient density. The recommendations on dietary fiber are based on proposed health benefits, such as reduced risk of several types of cancer, cardiovascular disease, type 2 diabetes, and obesity[61].

FOOD SOURCES

Food sources that contain primarily carbohydrates are cereals, bread, pasta, rice, fruit, vegetables, soft drinks, and sweets. The

GI and GL of products within these categories can vary a lot, depending on the amount of dietary fiber, the amount of carbohydrate, the degree of polymerization, and the food matrix. The ten food groups contributing to most carbohydrate intake in Europe are listed below in table 8[62]:

Table 8. This table illustrates the top 10 food items that contribute the most to the dietary carbohydrate intake in Europe. The numbers are the percentage of total carbohydrate intake.

Food item	Percentage contribution of total carbohydrate intake
Bread	26,6
Fruits	12,9
Milk and milk products	8,4
Potatoes	6,8
Sugar and jam	6,2
Sweet buns, cakes, and pies	7,3
Pasta and rice	6
Vegetables and legumes	4,1
Crispbread	2,9
Fruit and vegetable juices	2,8

(62)

PRACTICAL RECOMMENDATIONS FOR ESPORTS ATHLETES

If one is to sustain a good performance over several years in esports, it is crucial to focus not only on the acute performance aspect of nutritional interventions but also on long-term health. By following the recommendations mentioned earlier, one will most likely reduce the risk of diet-related diseases, such as diabetes mellitus, cardiovascular diseases, obesity, and different types of cancer. Adhering to these guidelines is important for general health but also the longevity of a potential esports career. Also, having many health issues might impact the quality of performance, both in the short and long term.

As for the recommended carbohydrate intake, a low intake (e.g., below 40% of the daily caloric intake) might impact the fiber and micronutrient intake, which might lead to impaired bowel function and micronutrient deficiencies. A very high carbohydrate intake (e.g., above 60% of total daily caloric intake) will impact the distribution of protein and fat, which might lead to deficiencies of certain essential amino acids or micronutrients that are exclusive to these macronutrients. Another risk, at least in the well-developed countries, is that the diet might contain too much sugar.

The carbohydrate intake should always be adjusted to individual demands. However, esports players, in general, do sit a lot during the day in order to practice. By default, this means that the general physical activity level will be low, even though there are exceptions to this assumption. A low physical activity level will lower the demand for carbohydrate in the diet but not below the recommended 40% of dietary intake as stated earlier because of its potential negative impact on essential nutrients. Esports players with an active lifestyle, training several days a week with high intensity, will need far more carbohydrate in the diet.

For competitive gaming, random spikes in blood sugar levels while playing are detrimental for performance. Therefore, minimizing the amount of sugar in the diet is essential. Some studies report the potential benefits of simple sugars and cognitive performance, but there is no consensus on this matter. If someone wants to try out these strategies, it is advisable to do this with a nutritionist. Also, the degree of negative impact consuming simple sugars can have on performance might outweigh the benefits.

On a more practical matter, the number of carbohydrates should be spread out evenly in the meals. Avoid vast amounts of carbohydrates in one meal, especially in meals before competitive play. This might lead to a substantial glycemic load, at least if the food items have a high glycemic index. As a result, one can end up with sub-optimally regulated blood sugar that will leave one feeling exhausted and unfocused during long competitive play.

The guidelines for carbohydrates for esports players can be summarized as follows:

1. Carbohydrate intake of 40% to 60% of total daily caloric intake
2. A minimum intake of 25 grams (women) and 35 grams (men) of dietary fiber per day
3. Choosing whole-grain products and vegetables for every meal
4. As low a sugar intake as possible, at least below 10% of the daily caloric intake
5. Carbohydrates spread out evenly in the meals (Avoid large amounts of carbohydrates in a meal.)

ALCOHOL

STRUCTURE AND FUNCTION

When alcohol (also known as ethanol) is oxidized in the body, the energy we get from it is approximately 7 kcal per gram. It is absorbed through passive diffusion primarily in the small intestine and is distributed to the total water content of the body[15]. The intake of ethanol can inhibit protein- and fat oxidation by up to 40% and 75% respectively. Its uptake is fairly quick and happens in the upper gastrointestinal tract. After 5 minutes, ethanol is present in the blood. The level of alcohol in the blood will depend on several factors: absorption rate, liver function, and pathophysiological factors. Most of it is oxidized in the body, but a small amount (<10%) is eliminated through urine and expiration. It is oxidized at a rate of 6 to 10 grams per hour. However, food still in the stomach will slow down the absorption of the alcohol, as well as dull the peak blood alcohol concentration. A meal rich in protein will blunt this response the most, which may be due to increased portal blood flow in response to feeding[21].

Alcohol has many detrimental effects on the human body when misused chronically, with 10-20% of abusers having cirrhosis, 30% having gastrointestinal problems, and 80% getting fatty liver. There are also strong associations between alcohol intake and an increased risk of different types of cancer[15; 21].

COGNITIVE PERFORMANCE

There are many studies on alcohol intake and cognitive performance, with most studies showing a clear detrimental effect. In speeded tasks, which are based on reaction time (e.g., a button press, it is commonly noted that the central stages (working memory and response selection) are negatively affected by alcohol consumption. Divided attention tasks, which can require both speed and precision, are negatively affected by alcohol as well. When an individual has to respond to two tasks (stimuli) at the same time (e.g., dodging a flashbang while trying to shoot back) within a close timeframe, this adverse effect of the alcohol leads to delayed response time to the second task[63].

Other tests that are used to determine cognitive function, and that can have applicability for esports athletes, are "inspection time", the "Traveling Salesperson Problem", the "Useful Field of View

Test" and the "Sustained Attention to Response Task." Most of these tests showed negative results for cognitive performance under the effect of alcohol[64].

GENERAL RECOMMENDATIONS

The Nordic Nutrition Recommendations 2012 recommend an alcohol intake below 10 grams per day for women, and below 20 grams per day for men[15]. However, the recommendations vary a lot between different countries. The recommendations usually range from 8 g per day up to 30 and 40 g, for women and men respectively[65].

FOOD SOURCES

Typical food sources that have a high content of alcohol are beer, wine, cider, sherry, and spirits. The table below shows different alcohol content in grams, as well as kcal per 100 ml of alcoholic beverage[21].

Table 9. The table shows different types of alcoholic beverages, with their respective kcal content, as well as alcohol amount in grams. Both kcal and alcohol are shown per 100 ml of alcoholic beverage.

Beverage	Kcal	Alcohol in grams
Alcohol-free lager	7	Trace amounts
Lager	29	4
Cider	36	3,8
Wine (red)	68	9,6
Wine (white, dry)	66	9,1
Sherry (dry)	116	15,7
Spirits (40% proof)	222	31,7

(21)

PRACTICAL RECOMMENDATIONS FOR ESPORTS ATHLETES

Esports competitors should be aware of any alcohol intake with regard to performance. The alcohol intake should be reduced to a minimum, as most of the scientific evidence indicates a reduced cognitive performance during or in the hours after intake. Also, clear evidence regarding its negative impact on health should be considered.

FLUID AND WATER INTAKE

About 45 to 75% of total body weight is water, muscle mass contains 70 to 75% water, and fat tissue water content varies between 10 and 40%. Water has vital functions in our body; e.g., it acts as a nutrient transporter, regulates body temperature, and provides cell and tissue structure[66].

During the day, the average fluid loss in a healthy adult is about 1,000 to 3,100 ml. This fluid loss is due to urinary excretion, fecal water output, respiratory water loss, and insensible water loss (e.g., sweating). Fluid intake is mostly through food and water but also from the oxidation of fat, protein, and carbohydrates[15; 66].

DEHYDRATION AND COGNITIVE PERFORMANCE

Avoiding dehydration is essential for esports players, as dehydration may cause a decline in cognitive performance. Most studies indicate a performance decline when dehydration is between 2 and 3% of total body weight[66; 67; 68; 69]. It also appears that the decline continues with increased dehydration[70]. Dehydration of more than 3 to 5% of body weight can reduce both endurance and strength, while dehydration of 15 to 25% of body weight can be fatal. There are no upper levels set for water intake;

however, acute water toxicity has been reported due to a water intake that exceeds the kidneys' maximal excretion rate[15].

Dehydration is common in athletes doing high-intensity training over a prolonged period, as well as athletes training or competing in a hot climate. Esports athletes do not face these same issues, but without proper nutrition and fluid intake over a prolonged period, dehydration can occur. Dehydration can arise from inadequate fluid intake or excessive fluid losses. One can also overhydrate, which is the case with excessive water/fluid intake or without a proper electrolyte replacement[71].

GENERAL RECOMMENDATIONS

The guiding value for fluid intake from the Nordic Nutrition Recommendations 2012 is 1 to 1,5 liters per day for ages 14 years and above. This recommended fluid intake comes in addition to the water from foods[15]. The Institute of Medicine recommends a total of 3000 and 2200 ml for men and women (age 19+) respectively, for total fluid intake, including water. For the age group 14 to 18 years, the recommendations are a bit lower: 1800 ml for females and 2600 ml for males[66]. The European Food Safety Authority (EFSA) recommends 2,000 ml for women and 2,500 ml for men as adequate intake[72].

PRACTICAL RECOMMENDATIONS FOR ESPORTS ATHLETES

As an esports player, one should use water as the go-to drink when feeling thirsty. Since one does not have any high physical demands in a hot climate, the fluid loss during gaming is quite low. The only thing that can influence this is if the competition is in a hot climate for a prolonged period. Also, if doing demanding physical training, like running, one should be aware of the increased fluid demands.

Therefore, most people meet the daily hydration needs based on thirst alone. An exact amount of recommended water per day is impossible to give, since daily needs may vary a lot, depending on physical activity and climate. Based on the recommendations above, drinking approximately ten glasses of water (1 glass equals 250 ml) should, in most cases, be enough to keep you hydrated.

FACTORS AFFECTING ESPORTS PERFORMANCE

SLEEP

Sleep is crucial for several biological functions, e.g., memory, learning, physiological processes, and cognitive function[73]. Sleep deprivation impacts hormonal levels, increasing the secretion of catabolic hormones[74] and cortisol[75]. Apart from harming performance, lack of sleep can have adverse health effects.

Sleep is separated into two distinct categories: rapid eye movement (REM) and non-rapid eye movement (NREM)[76]. Furthermore, NREM sleep is divided into four stages, each characterizing a deeper state of sleep. NREM sleep is also called slow wave sleep, characterized by its delta waves and high-voltage slow wave activity. This sleep is crucial for normal physical and intellectual performance and behavior[77]. REM sleep, however, is the sleep state in which we dream, with an electroencephalogram, resembling that of alert waking[78]. The functional role of REM sleep is still debated, but it is in this sleep we dream the most vivid dreams, and it is hypothesized that it is a critical factor in brain development[79].

SLEEP DEPRIVATION AND COGNITIVE PERFORMANCE

Cognitive performance in this sense is generally defined as goal-directed behavior requiring mental effort, which coincides with the basic requirements for esports athletes[76]. Sleep efficiency is known to be correlated with several critical cognitive functions, e.g., attention and concentration, sensory-perceptual function, memory, and executive and intellectual functions[80; 81]. These are all skills likely to be essential to perform at a top level as an esports athlete.

Mood also seems to be profoundly affected, even more so than performance[82]. A bad mood can, in turn, affect the individual player's performance. For esports athletes in a team, this can result in a negative atmosphere and a lousy performance for the whole group.

SLEEP DEPRIVATION AND HEALTH

Several studies report adverse health effects of sleep deprivation[76]. Chronic partial sleep loss can increase the risk of diabetes and obesity due to insulin resistance, increased energy intake, or dysregulation of the neuroendocrine control of appetite[83; 84]. Appetite-regulating hormones such as ghrelin and leptin are also affected by sleep deprivation, with an increased release of ghrelin, which increases the appetite. Leptin, the appetite-reducing hormone, is shown to be reduced when a person is sleep-deprived[85].

NUTRITIONAL INTERVENTIONS TO IMPROVE SLEEP

There are potential mechanisms to improve sleep with dietary intervention, in particular through neurotransmitters associated with the sleep-wake cycle. Some of these transmitters are 5-HT (serotonin), gamma-aminobutyric acid (GABA), noradrenaline, histamine, and orexin[86].

5-HT AND MELATONIN

The synthesis of 5-HT is dependent on the brain availability of L-tryptophan (Trp), which is the precursor of 5-HT. A strategy can, therefore, be to increase the Trp-levels through supplementation or dietary intervention, which, in turn, will lead to an increased concentration of 5-HT[76]. However, it is important to note that increasing the Trp-levels alone might not increase the 5-HT concentration if Trp is competing with other large, neutral amino acids. Therefore, the ratio between Trp and the other competing amino acids is essential. If 5-HT levels are to increase, the benefits could potentially be improved mood, behavior, sleep, and cognition. Currently, the three most effective ways to increase Trp-levels in the brain are through supplementation, increasing carbohydrate intake, or consuming proteins rich in Trp[87]. Good sources of protein with a high amount of Trp are meat, egg-whites, seafood, milk, dairy products, and cheese[88].

5-HT also serves as a precursor of melatonin, a hormone that has a sleep-inducing effect[89]. Ingestion of tart cherry juice concentrate has been shown to make modest improvements in sleep time and quality. It is supposed that tart cherry juice concentrate increases exogenous melatonin, which, in turn, improves sleep quality. The improved effect on sleep might be due to cytokines associated with the sleep-wake cycle, as the tart cherry juice is richer in both antioxidants and anti-inflammatory phytochemicals than the proposed melatonin[90].

CARBOHYDRATE

Some intervention studies are investigating the effect of carbohydrate intake on sleep quality and quantity[91; 92; 93; 94; 95]. One of these studies indicates that ingestion of high-glycemic carbohydrates before sleep might improve sleep quality and quantity[94]. Meals with a higher carbohydrate content rather than a lower carbohydrate content also seem to increase REM sleep, with decreased light sleep[95]. In contrast, one of the studies provided children with either a high-GI drink or a low-GI drink 1 hour before sleep. The group that was given the high-GI drink had increased arousal compared to the group with the low-GI drink[92]. One study looked at the food-matrix of meals, comparing solid versus liquid meals, and indicated that solid meals enhanced reduced sleep-onset latency (time to fall asleep)[91]. Finally, another looked at diet composition ("low-carb" vs. "high-carb") and found that the "low-carb" diet participants had increased deep sleep, while the "high-carb" participants had increased REM sleep[93]. Recommendations are difficult owing to the contradictory nature of these results, but there might be some positive effects of ingesting high-GI foods if consumed more than 1 hour before bedtime, as well as eating solid food rather than liquid food[76]. However, one should be aware of the potential negative consequences of ingesting high-GI food in considerable quantities in the long-term, as stated earlier. Usually, food items rich in carbohydrates with a high GI contain much sugar and few micronutrients.

MIXED MEALS AND DIET COMPOSITION

Only a few studies compare various mixed meals and diet composition and the effects on sleep[96; 97; 98; 99; 100; 101]. One study on mixed meals provided a drink with the evening meal, which consisted either of fat (90 g), carbohydrate (223 g) or protein (30 g). This study showed no effect on sleep between the different groups[97]. Low-calorie and high-calorie liquid meals before a day-time nap were compared to no meal, where both liquid meals showed increased sleep time in two sleep stages but with no difference in sleep-onset latency[96].

The studies on diet composition measured the effects on sleep after 4 to 7 days on a specific diet intervention, in contrast to many of the earlier studies that have been mentioned. One study showed an increased sleep latency on a low-carbohydrate (50 grams per day) diet for seven days, but the study included only six female subjects[100]. In a more extensive study, 44 adults, from 19 to 22 years old, were divided into four groups, with each group working as its own control group, and rotating between the four different diet compositions. The 4 diet intervention groups were high-protein (56% protein, 22% carbohydrate, and 22% fat), high-fat (56% fat, 22% carbohydrate, and 22% protein), high-carbohydrate (56% carbohydrate, 22% protein, and 22% fat) and a control diet (50% carbohydrate, 35% fat, and 15% protein)[98]. The high-protein diet showed fewer waking episodes during sleep, which might be due to the effects of Trp, as discussed earlier. The high-carbohydrate diets had a shorter sleep latency than the other diets, which is in contrast to another study that had two test meals, high-carbohydrate (15,5% protein, 12,5% fat, and 72% carbohydrate) and low carbohydrate (38% protein, 61% fat, and <1% carbohydrate)[93]. However, the sample size was low (14 participants), and the composition of the test meals differed in the two studies. To summarize, the research is currently inconclusive, but it is speculated that high-carbohydrate diets (>50% of TDEE) might reduce sleep latency, while high-protein diets may improve sleep quality[76; 102].

OTHER NUTRITIONAL INTERVENTIONS

While the literature is scarce regarding other sleep-promoting interventions, some foods might be beneficial. Fatty fish is a good source of vitamin D, as well as containing essential omega-3 fatty acids, which are essential for serotonin regulation. Also, food items such as kiwi and tart cherry juice, as mentioned earlier, might promote sleep quality. However, the studies are few; hence, it is difficult to give solid recommendations[102]. Substances or food items proposed to enhance sleep quality should be tailored to the individual in cooperation with a nutritionist or dietitian for best possible results.

PRACTICAL RECOMMENDATIONS FOR ESPORTS ATHLETES

Sleep is an essential factor for optimal performance as an esports athlete, as well as for health. Getting the right quality and quantity of sleep is not always easy, with a lot of practice or competitive play being in the afternoon and evening. Getting enough sleep can be a challenge if one must wake up early in the morning. The quality of sleep can also be affected when using media devices close to bedtime[103]. Interventions that might improve overall sleep are physical activity, reducing body weight (if being obese or overweight is causing obstructive sleep apnea), and reducing alcohol intake[104].

Besides the factors mentioned above, nutritional interventions might improve sleep. Some neurotransmitters are affected by what we eat. The following points might improve an athlete's sleep quality and quantity, but be aware that the literature is somewhat contradictory, and more studies are needed on this aspect of nutrition.

- Protein in the pre-sleep meal. Make sure the content of the amino acid Trp is high in the protein source (as in milk, cheese, egg whites, dairy products, meat, and seafood).
- Also, carbohydrate and fat sources with a high Trp content, such as potatoes, chickpeas, walnuts, hazelnuts, and cashew nuts, can be combined with the protein sources mentioned above to get a higher ratio of Trp in the meal.
- Tart cherry juice or milk with the evening meal.

- High GI-meals > 1 hour before sleep. However, be aware of potential health risks when using this strategy in combination with a high GL over time.
- Mixed meals might be the best, but the data is inconclusive. A combination of high amounts of carbohydrates (>50% of the energy from the meal) and Trp-rich protein seems to be better than other meal compositions.
- Other specific food categories that might improve sleep are fatty fish (omega-3 fatty acids) and fruits (kiwi, tart cherry juice).

ENERGY DRINKS

ENERGY DRINKS

By 2024, the size of the Global Energy Drink Market is estimated to reach a stunning 72 billion USD[105]. Energy drinks (EDs) are popular with young consumers, and the annual consumption exceeded 5,8 billion liters in approximately 160 countries in 2013[106]. A lot of the EDs sold contains caffeine in varying degrees. Most products range from 6 mg (decaffeinated) per serving up to 242 mg per serving. Even though the caffeine dose is stipulated on the label of the energy drink, it has been shown that it can vary a lot, even up to 20% higher than stated[107].

EDs also contain a lot of other bioactive substances such as taurine, L-carnitine, herbal supplements, inositol, and various B vitamins. These components will not be discussed here but are covered elsewhere[108]. EDs can also be sugar-dense, which can be detrimental for health, as mentioned earlier. Liquid carbohydrates do not provide any satiety, considering their food matrix. It is also easy to forget the negative impact these drinks have on the teeth[109]. It is a common problem when consuming a lot of EDs, with a probability of a 2,4-fold risk of dental erosion[110].

There are indications that long-term overuse of caffeine alone, and in combination with these bioactive substances found in Eds, may be harmful[106; 108]. Currently, there are no proven positive effects of the other bioactive substances in these drinks[108].

GENERAL RECOMMENDATIONS

The intake of EDs should not be above the recommended guidelines. The guidelines for caffeine are listed in the next section, "Caffeine."

FOOD SOURCES

Table 10 lists different EDs and some of their contents, per 16 oz (usually a can), unless mentioned otherwise.

Table 10. The table shows some of the most popular energy drinks and some of their nutritional content. The vitamins are as listed by the Food and Drug Administration as a percentage of daily value (DV) to help consumers compare nutrients of products in the context of a total diet.

Product	Sugar, mg	Caffeine, mg	Taurine, mg	Vitamin B$_6$, %DV	Vitamin B$_{12}$, %DV	Sodium, mg
Red bull	54	148	2000	480	Not listed	187
Monster Energy	54	173	Not listed	200	Not listed	360
Rock Star, Original	58	144	Listed, no amount given	320	Not listed	77
No Fear, Original	66	140	Listed as a proprietary blend	200	200	210
Full Throttle, Original	58	160	Not listed	200	200	160
NOS	53	160	Not listed	200	200	400

Data collected from manufacturers' website, 25. February 2019.

PRACTICAL RECOMMENDATIONS FOR ESPORTS ATHLETES

Even though EDs contain caffeine, and caffeine might be able to improve performance, the combination of all these substances in large amounts may have adverse health effects. Also, the other components in the ED do not have well-documented performance-enhancing effects. Because of this, one should not consume more than the general recommendations.

CAFFEINE

STRUCTURE AND FUNCTION

Caffeine, also called 1,3,7-trimethylxanthine, is similar to adenosine and has its ergogenic effect on our body through interactions with four receptors called A_1, A_{2a}, A_{2b}, and A_3. The receptor sensitivity and density can vary among individuals and are up-regulated as the caffeine intake increases[111]. Caffeine binds to these adenosine receptors that are located in the central and peripheral nervous systems, blood vessels, and organs such as the heart[112].

Caffeine is rapidly absorbed when ingested through food, drinks, or supplements. Within an hour, the caffeine reaches peak levels in the blood, however, with considerable individual variations[111]. Caffeine-containing gum is absorbed faster than the food items mentioned above, reaching peak levels within half the time compared with capsules. This is due to absorption through the buccal tissue of the mouth[113]. The half-life of caffeine is usually between 3 and 5 hours, although this can be affected by smoking, diseases, pregnancy, contraceptives, and diet[111]. It is metabolized by the enzyme CYP1A2 in the liver, by the cytochrome P450 oxidase enzyme system[112].

COGNITIVE PERFORMANCE

It has been well documented that caffeine affects several cognitive abilities, such as vigilance, wakefulness, and reaction time[112]. Two mechanisms might explain the effects of caffeine on performance. The first is an indirect and non-specific effect relating to arousal. This might explain why the effects of caffeine are more pronounced during sub-optimal conditions, such as sleep deprivation. The other mechanism is a more direct and specific effect, which relates to performance-enhancing effects such as improved perception, motor preparation, and execution[114]. In summary, caffeine seems to have a definite cognitive-enhancing effect on the abilities mentioned above, with the most pronounced effect on vigilance tasks and reaction time, both in rested and non-rested individuals[111].

GENERAL RECOMMENDATIONS

For the cognitive performance-enhancing effects, the proposed supplementation of caffeine ranges from 32 to 300 mg, or approximately 0,5 to 4 mg per kilo bodyweight[111]. However, the effective dosage depends on several factors, such as individual tolerance and regular dietary intake of caffeine. One should also note that too much caffeine can cause side-effects such as anxiety, nervousness, and jitteriness[112; 114]. This tolerance level is individual, but most cognitive performance-enhancing effects are seen at the levels mentioned earlier. Exceeding this level might cause more harm than good. Other side-effects that can appear when intoxicated are gastrointestinal disturbances, agitation, tremors, tachycardia, and, in some cases, death. The acute toxic level of caffeine is not well established yet, but some of the side-effects mentioned above may arise at intakes surpassing 500-600 mg[115].

For adults, the acute toxic effects of caffeine are proposed at approximately 10 grams per day[116].

Children and adolescents are more vulnerable to the effects of caffeine because of their lower body weight. These groups should be cautious when ingesting caffeine-rich products such as energy drinks[112]. An energy drink containing 80 mg caffeine (250 ml can), will give an adult weighing 80 kg a dose of 1 mg caffeine per kg body weight. However, a child weighing 30 kg will have an effective dose of almost 2,7 mg caffeine per kg body weight. EFSA has currently set the safety level at 3 mg per kg body weight per day[117].

FOOD SOURCES

Many foods and drinks, such as tea, soft drinks, chocolate, and energy drinks, contain caffeine. The caffeine from coffee and tea comes from their beans or leaves, while the caffeine in energy drinks is usually derived from guarana leaves. It also occurs naturally in cocoa, so it is found in chocolate. That means chocolate with higher amounts of cocoa contains more caffeine than chocolate with less cocoa[112]. Table 11 shows a list of food and drink items containing caffeine.

Table 11. The table illustrates different food items containing caffeine (mg) per 100 grams.

Food or drink	Caffeine per 100 grams, mg
100% cocoa chocolate	240
55% cocoa chocolate	124
33% cocoa chocolate (milk chocolate)	45
Coffee, regular filter	50 – 60
Espresso	120

Tea	26
Coca Cola and similar drinks	15
Energy drinks	35 - 66

(106; 118; 119)

PRACTICAL RECOMMENDATIONS FOR ESPORTS ATHLETES

For esports athletes, some abilities are arguably more important than others. Factors such as reaction time, vigilance, and wakefulness can be crucial in particular settings. Caffeine can promote some of these effects, but an over-use might be detrimental for both health and performance. The intake of caffeine should be tailored to the individual with the help of an expert, to achieve the best possible effect on cognitive performance. However, as a general guideline, an intake of 0,5 to 4 mg per kg body weight approximately 15 to 60 minutes before the competition might give the best effect, depending on the source of caffeine.

NOOTROPICS

WHAT ARE NOOTROPICS?

Nootropics are known by various names, such as "smart drugs," "brain boosters" or "memory-enhancing drugs"[120]. The definition of nootropics is compounds that boost several mental functions, e.g., memory, attention, concentration, and motivation. However, there is no consensus regarding nootropics' effect as a performance enhancer on young, healthy minds[121]. Another issue is the potential doping risk for esports athletes, as some dietary supplements and nootropics might contain illegal ingredients. Also, it is uncertain whether long-term use of certain nootropics might have unhealthy consequences[121; 122]. It is evident that the research in this field is expanding, as is the interest in their performance-enhancing abilities from both athletes and manufacturers.

PRACTICAL RECOMMENDATIONS FOR ESPORTS ATHLETES

Currently, no evidence recommends the usage of nootropics in a performance-enhancing setting for esports athletes. As stated earlier, there are health and doping risks when ingesting nootropics, so for the time being, abstaining from nootropics is the recommendation.

CONCLUSION

Nutrition in esports is still in its infancy, but there exist some guidelines that apply to both gamers and esports athletes. The scope of this book is to enlighten everyone interested in this topic, as well as give both gamers and esports athletes some practical advice they can apply to their diet to improve both health and performance. It is important to emphasize the importance of health in relation to acute performance, as well as the longevity of the esports career. Esports involves a lot of dedication and practice, requiring the athletes to sit for extended periods. Having a healthy diet, as well as regular physical activity, will most certainly be beneficial for health and performance to help counter-balance the adverse effects of this sedentary lifestyle.

As with other sports, there are no shortcuts to achieving high performance. By that, I mean no vitamin, mineral, performance-enhancing substance or specific food will make you perform ten times better, even though some of the potential dietary interventions proposed in this book might improve your performance marginally. It is essential to understand that adhering to the general guidelines for a healthy diet will be the "bread and butter" for your health and performance.

So, if you want to make the best out of your esports career – why not start by improving your diet?

REFERENCES

1. Seth E. Jenny RDM, Margaret C. Keiper & Tracy W. Olrich (2016) Virtual(ly) Athletes: Where eSports Fit Within the Definition of "Sport". *Quest* **69**, 1-18.

2. Esports NAoC (2019) School Directory. https://nacesports.org/school-directory/ (accessed 04.03.2019)

3. Conditt J (2018) College esports is set to explode, starting with the Fiesta Bowl. https://www.engadget.com/2018/02/22/college-esports-is-set-to-explode-starting-with-the-fiesta-bowl/ (accessed 04.03.2019)

4. Newzoo (2019) Esports awareness exceeds 1 billion as new global & local initiatives are launched. https://newzoo.com/insights/articles/global-esports-awareness-exceeds-1-billion-as-new-initiatives-launched/ (accessed 09.01.2019)

5. Statista (2019) eSports audience size worldwide from 2012 to 2022, by type of viewers (in millions). https://www.statista.com/statistics/490480/global-esports-audience-size-viewer-type/ (accessed 04.03.2019)

6. Banyai F, Griffiths MD, Kiraly O *et al.* (2018) The Psychology of Esports: A Systematic Literature Review. *J Gambl Stud.*

7. Campbell MJ, Toth AJ, Moran AP *et al.* (2018) eSports: A new window on neurocognitive expertise? *Prog Brain Res* **240**, 161-174.

8. Choi C, Hums MA, Bum CH (2018) Impact of the Family Environment on Juvenile Mental Health: eSports Online Game Addiction and Delinquency. *Int J Environ Res Public Health* **15**.

9. DiFrancisco-Donoghue J, Balentine J, Schmidt G *et al.* (2019) Managing the health of the eSport athlete: an integrated health management model. *BMJ Open Sport Exerc Med* **5**, e000467.

10. Peter SC, Li Q, Pfund RA *et al.* (2018) Public Stigma Across Addictive Behaviors: Casino Gambling, eSports Gambling, and Internet Gaming. *J Gambl Stud.*

11. Statista (2017) Number of active video gamers worldwide from 2014 to 2021 (in millions). https://www.statista.com/statistics/748044/number-video-gamers-world/ (accessed 11.01.2019)

12. Statista (2017) Distribution of video gamers worldwide in 2017, by age group and gender. https://www.statista.com/statistics/722259/world-gamers-by-age-and-gender/ (accessed 10.01.2019)

13. USDA (2002) *USDoA: Profiling Food Consumption in America.*

14. Myles IA (2014) Fast food fever: reviewing the impacts of the Western diet on immunity. *Nutr J* **13**, 61.

15. NNR (2012) Nordic Nutrition Recommendations 2012. In *Integrating Nutrition and Physical Activity*, 5th ed.

16. Hills AP, Mokhtar N, Byrne NM (2014) Assessment of physical activity and energy expenditure: an overview of objective measures. *Front Nutr* **1**, 5.

17. Organization FAA (2001) Human energy requirements. *Report of a Joint FAO/WHO/UNU Expert Consultation.* http://www.fao.org/docrep/007/Y5686E/y5686e07.htm

18. Khan SS, Ning H, Wilkins JT *et al.* (2018) Association of Body Mass Index With Lifetime Risk of Cardiovascular Disease and Compression of Morbidity. *JAMA Cardiol* **3**, 280-287.

19. Illner K, Brinkmann G, Heller M *et al.* (2000) Metabolically active components of fat free mass and resting energy expenditure in nonobese adults. *Am J Physiol Endocrinol Metab* **278**, E308-315.

20. Nelson KM, Weinsier RL, Long CL *et al.* (1992) Prediction of resting energy expenditure from fat-free mass and fat mass. *Am J Clin Nutr* **56**, 848-856.

21. Geissler C, Powers H. (2005) *Human Nutrition.* 11th ed: Elsevier, Churchill Livingstone.

22. Foure A, Bendahan D (2017) Is Branched-Chain Amino Acids Supplementation an Efficient Nutritional Strategy to Alleviate Skeletal Muscle Damage? A Systematic Review. *Nutrients* **9**.

23. Wolfe RR (2017) Branched-chain amino acids and muscle protein synthesis in humans: myth or reality? *J Int Soc Sports Nutr* **14**, 30.

24. Hoffman JR, Falvo MJ (2004) Protein - Which is Best? *J Sports Sci Med* **3**, 118-130.

25. Schaafsma G (2005) The Protein Digestibility-Corrected Amino Acid Score (PDCAAS) – a concept for describing protein quality in foods and food ingredients: a critical review. *J AOAC Int* **88**, 988-994.

26. Phillips SM (2014) A brief review of critical processes in exercise-induced muscular hypertrophy. *Sports Med* **44 Suppl 1**, S71-77.

27. Lonnie M, Hooker E, Brunstrom JM *et al.* (2018) Protein for Life: Review of Optimal Protein Intake, Sustainable Dietary Sources and the Effect on Appetite in Ageing Adults. *Nutrients* **10**.

28. WHO (2002) Protein and amino acid requirements in human nutrition.

29. Churchward-Venne TA, Burd NA, Phillips SM (2012) Nutritional regulation of muscle protein synthesis with resistance exercise: strategies to enhance anabolism. *Nutr Metab (Lond)* **9**, 40.

30. Burke LD, Vicki (2010) *Clinical Sports Nutrition.* Fourth ed: McGraw-Hill Australia Pty Ltd.

31. Stokes T, Hector AJ, Morton RW *et al.* (2018) Recent Perspectives Regarding the Role of Dietary Protein for the Promotion of Muscle Hypertrophy with Resistance Exercise Training. *Nutrients* **10**.

32. Young VR, Pellett PL (1994) Plant proteins in relation to human protein and amino acid nutrition. *Am J Clin Nutr* **59**, 1203S-1212S.

33. (FAO) FaAO (2010) The State of Food Insecurity in the World, Addressing Food Insecurity in Protracted Crisis.

34. Blesso CN, Fernandez ML (2018) Dietary Cholesterol, Serum Lipids, and Heart Disease: Are Eggs Working for or Against You? *Nutrients* **10**.

35. Cohn JS, Kamili A, Wat E *et al.* (2010) Dietary phospholipids and intestinal cholesterol absorption. *Nutrients* **2**, 116-127.

36. Kremmyda LS, Tvrzicka E, Stankova B *et al.* (2011) Fatty acids as biocompounds: their role in human metabolism, health and disease: a review. part 2: fatty acid physiological roles and applications in human health and disease. *Biomed Pap Med Fac Univ Palacky Olomouc Czech Repub* **155**, 195-218.

37. Zock PL, Blom WA, Nettleton JA *et al.* (2016) Progressing Insights into the Role of Dietary Fats in the Prevention of Cardiovascular Disease. *Curr Cardiol Rep* **18**, 111.

38. Allaire J, Couture P, Leclerc M *et al.* (2016) A randomized, crossover, head-to-head comparison of eicosapentaenoic acid and docosahexaenoic acid supplementation to reduce inflammation markers in men and women: the Comparing

EPA to DHA (ComparED) Study. *Am J Clin Nutr* **104**, 280-287.

39. Chang CL, Deckelbaum RJ (2013) Omega-3 fatty acids: mechanisms underlying 'protective effects' in atherosclerosis. *Curr Opin Lipidol* **24**, 345-350.

40. Mozaffarian D, Geelen A, Brouwer IA *et al.* (2005) Effect of fish oil on heart rate in humans: a meta-analysis of randomized controlled trials. *Circulation* **112**, 1945-1952.

41. Miller PE, Van Elswyk M, Alexander DD (2014) Long-chain omega-3 fatty acids eicosapentaenoic acid and docosahexaenoic acid and blood pressure: a meta-analysis of randomized controlled trials. *Am J Hypertens* **27**, 885-896.

42. Musa-Veloso K, Binns MA, Kocenas AC *et al.* (2010) Long-chain omega-3 fatty acids eicosapentaenoic acid and docosahexaenoic acid dose-dependently reduce fasting serum triglycerides. *Nutr Rev* **68**, 155-167.

43. Dyall SC (2015) Long-chain omega-3 fatty acids and the brain: a review of the independent and shared effects of EPA, DPA and DHA. *Front Aging Neurosci* **7**, 52.

44. Abubakari AR, Naderali MM, Naderali EK (2014) Omega-3 fatty acid supplementation and cognitive function: are smaller dosages more beneficial? *Int J Gen Med* **7**, 463-473.

45. Mazereeuw G, Lanctot KL, Chau SA *et al.* (2012) Effects of omega-3 fatty acids on cognitive performance: a meta-analysis. *Neurobiol Aging* **33**, 1482 e1417-1429.

46. Rangel-Huerta OD, Gil A (2018) Effect of omega-3 fatty acids on cognition: an updated systematic review of randomized clinical trials. *Nutr Rev* **76**, 1-20.

47. Bauer I, Hughes M, Rowsell R *et al.* (2014) Omega-3 supplementation improves cognition and modifies brain activation in young adults. *Hum Psychopharmacol* **29**, 133-144.

48. FAO (2010) Fats and fatty acids in human nutrition.

49. Health NIo (2018) Omega-3 Fatty Acids. *Fact Sheet for Health Professionals.* https://ods.od.nih.gov/factsheets/Omega3FattyAcids-HealthProfessional/ (accessed 28.01.2019)

50. Mattilsynet (2019) Matvaretabellen. http://www.matvaretabellen.no/ (accessed 28.01.2019)

51. Möller's Tran. https://www.mollers.no/produkt/mollers-tran/ (accessed 29.01.2019

52. Belorkar SA, Gupta AK (2016) Oligosaccharides: a boon from nature's desk. *AMB Express* **6**, 82.

53. Nantle G (1998) Carbohydrates in human nutrition.

54. Lambo AM, Öste, R., Nyman, M.E.G. (2004) Dietary fibre in fermented oat and barley β- glucan rich concentrates. *Food Chemistry* **89**, 283-293.

55. Dhingra D, Michael M, Rajput H *et al.* (2012) Dietary fibre in foods: a review. *J Food Sci Technol* **49**, 255-266.

56. Liu S, Manson JE (2001) Dietary carbohydrates, physical inactivity, obesity, and the 'metabolic syndrome' as predictors of coronary heart disease. *Curr Opin Lipidol* **12**, 395-404.

57. Nehir ES (1999) Determination of glycemic index for some breads.

58. Russell WR, Baka A, Bjorck I *et al.* (2016) Impact of Diet Composition on Blood Glucose Regulation. *Crit Rev Food Sci Nutr* **56**, 541-590.

59. Hawkins MAW, Keirns NG, Helms Z (2018) Carbohydrates and cognitive function. *Curr Opin Clin Nutr Metab Care* **21**, 302-307.

60. Buyken AE, Mela DJ, Dussort P *et al.* (2018) Dietary carbohydrates: a review of international recommendations

and the methods used to derive them. *Eur J Clin Nutr* **72**, 1625-1643.

61. Helsedirektoratet (2018) Kostråd om grove kornprodukter. https://helsenorge.no/kosthold-og-ernaring/kostrad/spis-grove-kornprodukter (accessed 30.01.2019)

62. Wirfalt E, McTaggart A, Pala V *et al.* (2002) Food sources of carbohydrates in a European cohort of adults. *Public Health Nutr* **5**, 1197-1215.

63. Fillmore MT (2007) Acute alcohol-induced impairment of cognitive functions: Past and present findings.

64. Dry MJ, Burns NR, Nettelbeck T *et al.* (2012) Dose-related effects of alcohol on cognitive functioning. *PLoS One* **7**, e50977.

65. (IARD) IAfRD (2018) Drinking guidelines: General population. http://www.iard.org/resources/drinking-guidelines-general-population/

66. Riebl SK, Davy BM (2013) The Hydration Equation: Update on Water Balance and Cognitive Performance. *ACSMs Health Fit J* **17**, 21-28.

67. Wittbrodt MT, Millard-Stafford M (2018) Dehydration Impairs Cognitive Performance: A Meta-analysis. *Med Sci Sports Exerc* **50**, 2360-2368.

68. Adan A (2012) Cognitive performance and dehydration. *J Am Coll Nutr* **31**, 71-78.

69. Lieberman HR (2007) Hydration and cognition: a critical review and recommendations for future research. *J Am Coll Nutr* **26**, 555S-561S.

70. Pross N, Demazieres A, Girard N *et al.* (2013) Influence of progressive fluid restriction on mood and physiological markers of dehydration in women. *Br J Nutr* **109**, 313-321.

71. Montain SJ, Cheuvront SN, Sawka MN (2006) Exercise associated hyponatraemia: quantitative analysis to understand the aetiology. *Br J Sports Med* **40**, 98-105; discussion 198-105.

72. Authority EFS (2010) Scientific Opinion on Dietary Reference Values for water.

73. Cirelli C, Tononi G (2008) Is sleep essential? *PLoS Biol* **6**, e216.

74. Dattilo M, Antunes HK, Medeiros A *et al.* (2011) Sleep and muscle recovery: endocrinological and molecular basis for a new and promising hypothesis. *Med Hypotheses* **77**, 220-222.

75. Spiegel K, Leproult R, Van Cauter E (1999) Impact of sleep debt on metabolic and endocrine function. *Lancet* **354**, 1435-1439.

76. Halson SL (2014) Sleep in elite athletes and nutritional interventions to enhance sleep. *Sports Med* **44 Suppl 1**, S13-23.

77. de Andres I, Garzon M, Reinoso-Suarez F (2011) Functional Anatomy of Non-REM Sleep. *Front Neurol* **2**, 70.

78. Siegel JM (2005) *Principles and Practice of Sleep Medicine.* 4th ed.

79. Peever J, Fuller PM (2017) The Biology of REM Sleep. *Curr Biol* **27**, R1237-R1248.

80. Walker MP (2009) The role of sleep in cognition and emotion. *Ann N Y Acad Sci* **1156**, 168-197.

81. Deak MC, Stickgold R (2010) Sleep and cognition. *Wiley Interdiscip Rev Cogn Sci* **1**, 491-500.

82. Pilcher JJ, Huffcutt AI (1996) Effects of sleep deprivation on performance: a meta-analysis. *Sleep* **19**, 318-326.

83. Spiegel K, Knutson K, Leproult R *et al.* (2005) Sleep loss: a novel risk factor for insulin resistance and Type 2 diabetes. *J Appl Physiol (1985)* **99**, 2008-2019.

84. Knutson KL, Spiegel K, Penev P *et al.* (2007) The metabolic consequences of sleep deprivation. *Sleep Med Rev* **11**, 163-178.

85. Van Cauter E, Spiegel K, Tasali E *et al.* (2008) Metabolic consequences of sleep and sleep loss. *Sleep Med* **9 Suppl 1**, S23-28.

86. Saper CB, Scammell TE, Lu J (2005) Hypothalamic regulation of sleep and circadian rhythms. *Nature* **437**, 1257-1263.

87. Silber BY, Schmitt JA (2010) Effects of tryptophan loading on human cognition, mood, and sleep. *Neurosci Biobehav Rev* **34**, 387-407.

88. Palego L, Betti L, Rossi A *et al.* (2016) Tryptophan Biochemistry: Structural, Nutritional, Metabolic, and Medical Aspects in Humans. *J Amino Acids* **2016**, 8952520.

89. Klein DC, Moore RY (1979) Pineal N-acetyltransferase and hydroxyindole-O-methyltransferase: control by the retinohypothalamic tract and the suprachiasmatic nucleus. *Brain Res* **174**, 245-262.

90. Howatson G, Bell PG, Tallent J *et al.* (2012) Effect of tart cherry juice (Prunus cerasus) on melatonin levels and enhanced sleep quality. *Eur J Nutr* **51**, 909-916.

91. Orr WC, Shadid G, Harnish MJ *et al.* (1997) Meal composition and its effect on postprandial sleepiness. *Physiol Behav* **62**, 709-712.

92. Jalilolghadr S, Afaghi A, O'Connor H *et al.* (2011) Effect of low and high glycaemic index drink on sleep pattern in children. *J Pak Med Assoc* **61**, 533-536.

93. Afaghi A, O'Connor H, Chow CM (2008) Acute effects of the very low carbohydrate diet on sleep indices. *Nutr Neurosci* **11**, 146-154.

94. Afaghi A, O'Connor H, Chow CM (2007) High-glycemic-index carbohydrate meals shorten sleep onset. *Am J Clin Nutr* **85**, 426-430.

95. Porter JM, Horne JA (1981) Bed-time food supplements and sleep: effects of different carbohydrate levels. *Electroencephalogr Clin Neurophysiol* **51**, 426-433.

96. Zammit GK, Kolevzon A, Fauci M *et al.* (1995) Postprandial sleep in healthy men. *Sleep* **18**, 229-231.

97. Hartmann MK, Crisp AH, Evans G *et al.* (1979) Short-term effects of CHO, fat and protein loads on total tryptophan/tyrosine levels in plasma as related to %REM sleep. *Waking Sleeping* **3**, 63-68.

98. Lindseth G, Lindseth P, Thompson M (2013) Nutritional effects on sleep. *West J Nurs Res* **35**, 497-513.

99. Lacey JH, Hawkins C, Crisp AH (1978) Effects of dietary protein on sleep E.E.G. in normal subjects. *Adv Biosci* **21**, 245-247.

100. Kwan RM, Thomas S, Mir MA (1986) Effects of a low carbohydrate isoenergetic diet on sleep behavior and pulmonary functions in healthy female adult humans. *J Nutr* **116**, 2393-2402.

101. Grandner MA, Kripke DF, Naidoo N *et al.* (2010) Relationships among dietary nutrients and subjective sleep, objective sleep, and napping in women. *Sleep Med* **11**, 180-184.

102. St-Onge MP, Mikic A, Pietrolungo CE (2016) Effects of Diet on Sleep Quality. *Adv Nutr* **7**, 938-949.

103. Carter B, Rees, P., Hale, L. & Bhattacharjee, D. (2016) A meta-analysis of the effect of media devices on sleep outcomes.

104. Shochat T (2012) Impact of lifestyle and technology developments on sleep. *Nat Sci Sleep* **4**, 19-31.

105. Markets RA (2018) Global Energy Drink Market Analysis (2018-2024).

106. Alsunni AA (2015) Energy Drink Consumption: Beneficial and Adverse Health Effects. *Int J Health Sci (Qassim)* **9**, 468-474.

107. magazine CR (2012) The Buzz on Energy-Drink Caffeine. Caffeine Levels per Serving for the 27 Products We Checked Ranged from 6 Milligrams to 242 Milligrams per Serving.

108. Higgins JP, Tuttle TD, Higgins CL (2010) Energy beverages: content and safety. *Mayo Clin Proc* **85**, 1033-1041.

109. Bailey RL, Saldanha LG, Dwyer JT (2014) Estimating caffeine intake from energy drinks and dietary supplements in the United States. *Nutr Rev* **72 Suppl 1**, 9-13.

110. Li H, Zou Y, Ding G (2012) Dietary factors associated with dental erosion: a meta-analysis. *PLoS One* **7**, e42626.

111. McLellan TM, Caldwell JA, Lieberman HR (2016) A review of caffeine's effects on cognitive, physical and occupational performance. *Neurosci Biobehav Rev* **71**, 294-312.

112. Temple JL, Bernard C, Lipshultz SE *et al.* (2017) The Safety of Ingested Caffeine: A Comprehensive Review. *Front Psychiatry* **8**, 80.

113. Kamimori GH, Karyekar CS, Otterstetter R *et al.* (2002) The rate of absorption and relative bioavailability of caffeine administered in chewing gum versus capsules to normal healthy volunteers. *Int J Pharm* **234**, 159-167.

114. Nehlig A (2010) Is caffeine a cognitive enhancer? *J Alzheimers Dis* **20 Suppl 1**, S85-94.

115. Cappelletti S, Piacentino D, Sani G *et al.* (2015) Caffeine: cognitive and physical performance enhancer or psychoactive drug? *Curr Neuropharmacol* **13**, 71-88.

116. Greden JF (1974) Anxiety or caffeinism: a diagnostic dilemma. *Am J Psychiatry* **131**, 1089-1092.

117. Authority EFS (2015) Caffeine. *EFSA explains risk assessment.*

118. Folkehelseinstituttet (2015) Fakta om koffein og koffeinholdige drikker. https://www.fhi.no/ml/kosthold/fakta-om-koffein/#koffein-i-mat-og-drikke (accessed 26.02.2019)

119. Muller C, Vetter F, Richter E *et al.* (2014) Determination of caffeine, myosmine, and nicotine in chocolate by headspace solid-phase microextraction coupled with gas chromatography-tandem mass spectrometry. *J Food Sci* **79**, T251-255.

120. Suliman NA, Mat Taib CN, Mohd Moklas MA *et al.* (2016) Establishing Natural Nootropics: Recent Molecular Enhancement Influenced by Natural Nootropic. *Evid Based Complement Alternat Med* **2016**, 4391375.

121. Lanni C, Lenzken SC, Pascale A *et al.* (2008) Cognition enhancers between treating and doping the mind. *Pharmacol Res* **57**, 196-213.

122. Farah MJ, Illes J, Cook-Deegan R *et al.* (2004) Neurocognitive enhancement: what can we do and what should we do? *Nat Rev Neurosci* **5**, 421-425.